WALL PILATES FOR SENIORS

A Gentle Path to Vitality, Balance,
and Joyful Aging

JULIANNE CARRIE

DISCLAIMER

The information provided in this book is for educational and informational purposes only. It is not intended as a substitute for professional medical advice, diagnosis, or treatment. Always seek the advice of your physician or other qualified healthcare provider with any questions you may have regarding a medical condition or treatment.

The content of this book is based on general knowledge and research available up to the time of its publication. Health and medical information are subject to constant advancements and changes. Therefore, the author, publisher, and any contributors to this book make no representations or warranties of any kind, express or implied, regarding the accuracy, completeness, suitability, or applicability of the information contained herein.

Readers are encouraged to consult their healthcare providers before making any changes to their diet, exercise routines, or medical treatment plans. Individual responses to dietary and lifestyle changes can vary, and what works for one person may not work for another.

The author and publisher of this book are not responsible for any adverse effects, injuries, or damages arising from the information provided within these pages. Any reliance you place on the information in this book is strictly at your own risk.

Please consult your healthcare provider before beginning any new dietary or exercise program, making changes to your existing treatment plan, or relying on the information presented in this book. Your healthcare provider is the best source of information regarding your individual health situation.

By reading and utilizing the information in this book, you agree to the terms of this disclaimer.

If you do not agree with these terms, please refrain from using this book.

Remember that the field of health and medicine is complex and rapidly evolving. The information in this book is not a substitute for professional medical advice, and readers should always prioritize their health and safety by consulting qualified healthcare professionals.

TABLE OF CONTENT

Introduction

Welcome to the transformative world of Wall Pilates for Seniors! This guide is your key to unlocking a rejuvenating and empowering journey towards better health and vitality. Designed with the unique needs of seniors in mind, our Wall Pilates program offers a gentle yet highly effective approach to fitness.

Discover a New Dimension of Wellness

Are you ready to redefine your sense of well-being? Wall Pilates for Seniors is not just a workout; it's an invitation to embrace strength, flexibility, and balance in a way that harmonizes with the wisdom of aging. Say goodbye to conventional exercise routines and hello to a holistic approach that caters specifically to the needs of your body, mind, and spirit.

Why Wall Pilates?

As we age, staying active becomes more crucial than ever. Wall Pilates provides a low-impact solution that is not only gentle on joints but also incredibly effective in promoting muscle tone, flexibility, and core strength. By incorporating the support of a wall, we've created a program that allows you to focus on the joy of movement without the fear of strain.

What Awaits You Inside

In the following pages, you'll find a comprehensive guide to Wall Pilates for Seniors. From setting up your Pilates space to mastering advanced techniques, we've crafted a resource that caters to all fitness levels. Whether you're a newcomer to Pilates or a seasoned practitioner, our guide offers a variety of exercises and routines that can be tailored to your individual needs.

Embark on this journey with us, and let the walls become your allies in achieving a healthier, more vibrant you. It's time to embrace the benefits of Wall Pilates for Seniors and rediscover the joy of movement at any age.

Your well-being is worth the investment. Let's begin.

Purpose of the Guide

"Wall Pilates for Seniors" is more than just a compilation of exercises; it's a comprehensive guide with a clear and meaningful purpose. Let's delve into the multifaceted reasons behind the creation of this guide, ensuring you understand the depth of its intent and the value it brings to your wellness journey.

1. Empowering Seniors on Their Fitness Odyssey

The primary objective is to empower seniors on their unique fitness odyssey. Aging should not be a barrier to vitality; it should be a catalyst for resilience and strength. This guide is meticulously designed to provide seniors with the tools, knowledge, and inspiration to navigate their fitness journey with confidence, addressing the specific needs and nuances that come with age.

2. Holistic Wellness Integration

We embrace a holistic approach that extends beyond the physical. "Wall Pilates for Seniors" is crafted to enrich not only your body but also your mind and spirit. The incorporation of a supportive wall serves as a metaphorical foundation for a balanced and holistic well-being. Through mindful exercises, breathing techniques, and mental focus, we aim to elevate your fitness experience to a state of comprehensive wellness.

3. Inclusivity and Accessibility

Fitness is a universal right, and this guide is dedicated to making it accessible to every senior, regardless of their fitness level. Whether you're a beginner or have been practicing Pilates for years, our guide offers a range of exercises and routines tailored to meet you where you are. We believe in the inclusivity of fitness, and "Wall Pilates for Seniors" serves as a welcoming gateway to a healthier and more active lifestyle.

4. Sustainable Health Practices

Sustainability is key to lasting well-being. This guide is not about quick fixes; it's about cultivating sustainable health practices that become an integral part of your daily life. By providing diverse exercises, routines, and valuable insights, we aim to inspire a commitment to consistency and longevity in your fitness journey. "Wall Pilates for Seniors" is designed to be a lifelong companion, supporting your well-being through the years.

5. Fostering a Joyful and Fulfilling Experience

Fitness should be enjoyable, and this guide is crafted to make your Pilates experience joyful and fulfilling. We want you to look forward to your workouts, finding satisfaction in every movement. By incorporating a variety of exercises and routines, we aim to keep your fitness routine dynamic, engaging, and tailored to your preferences.

As you embark on this guide, keep these purposes in mind. It's not just about exercise; it's about embracing a holistic and empowering approach to senior fitness.

Benefits of Wall Pilates for Seniors

"Wall Pilates for Seniors" is a holistic fitness approach tailored to meet the unique needs of older adults. Discover the myriad benefits that make this program a transformative and enriching experience for seniors.

1. Gentle on Joints, Powerful on Muscles

Joint-Friendly: The support of a wall reduces impact on joints, making Wall Pilates a gentle yet effective option for seniors, promoting flexibility and mobility without strain.

Muscle Strengthening: Engage in low-impact resistance exercises that target key muscle groups, enhancing strength without compromising joint health.

2. Improved Posture and Balance
Postural Awareness: Wall Pilates emphasizes core engagement, contributing to improved posture and spinal alignment, crucial for preventing age-related postural issues.

Enhanced Balance: Specific exercises focus on balance and stability, reducing the risk of falls and promoting a confident and steady gait.

3. Mind-Body Connection

Mindful Movement: Wall Pilates encourages mindfulness in movement, fostering a deep mind-body connection that enhances coordination and cognitive function.

Stress Reduction: Incorporate breathing techniques and focused exercises that promote relaxation, reducing stress levels and promoting mental well-being.

4. Adaptable to Individual Needs
Customizable Routines: Tailor your Wall Pilates routine to your individual fitness level and specific needs, making it accessible and beneficial for seniors with varying abilities.

Modifications: Every exercise can be modified to accommodate any physical limitations or challenges, ensuring a safe and personalized fitness experience.

5. Enhanced Flexibility and Range of Motion
Dynamic Stretching: Wall Pilates includes dynamic stretching exercises that enhance flexibility and promote a full range of motion, vital for maintaining mobility as you age.

Joint Health: By promoting flexibility, Wall Pilates contributes to joint health, reducing stiffness and supporting overall joint function.

6. Social and Emotional Well-Being
Community Connection: Joining classes or practicing Wall Pilates in a group setting fosters a sense of community, reducing

feelings of isolation and promoting social well-being.

Positive Mindset: Regular physical activity, such as Wall Pilates, is linked to improved mood and a positive outlook, contributing to emotional well-being.

7. Accessible Anytime, Anywhere
Convenience: With minimal equipment and the adaptability of wall support, Wall Pilates can be practiced in the comfort of your home, promoting consistency and adherence to your fitness routine.

No Age Limit: Whether you're a newcomer to fitness or have been active throughout your life, Wall Pilates is suitable for seniors of all ages and fitness backgrounds.

Experience the holistic benefits of Wall Pilates for Seniors and embark on a journey to a healthier, more vibrant, and fulfilling life.

Understanding Wall Pilates

Welcome to the foundation of your fitness journey—Wall Pilates. This section is dedicated to providing a comprehensive understanding of what Wall Pilates is, its principles, and why it stands as a unique and effective fitness modality for seniors.

1. What is Pilates?

Pilates is a holistic fitness approach developed by Joseph Pilates that focuses on strengthening the core, improving flexibility, and promoting overall body awareness. It combines controlled movements with breath awareness to enhance physical and mental well-being.

2. Why Wall Pilates for Seniors?

Support and Stability: Wall Pilates introduces the use of a wall for support, providing stability and allowing seniors to perform exercises with confidence, especially beneficial for those with balance concerns.

Gentle yet Effective: Tailored to the specific needs of seniors, Wall Pilates offers a gentle, low-impact alternative that prioritizes joint health while still delivering a powerful workout for muscle strength and flexibility.

Adaptable to All Levels: Whether you're a beginner or a seasoned practitioner, Wall Pilates can be adapted to suit your individual fitness level, making it an inclusive and accessible option for all seniors.

3. The Core Principles of Wall Pilates

Centering: Emphasis on the core as the focal point of all movements, promoting stability and strength from the center outward.

Control: Mindful and controlled movements to engage specific muscle groups, fostering precision and awareness in each exercise.

Breathing: Coordinated breath with movement to enhance oxygen flow, reduce stress, and promote a sense of calm and focus.

Flow: Fluidity in transitions between movements, creating a seamless and connected exercise experience.

4. The Role of the Wall

Supportive Element: The wall serves as a supportive element, offering a stable surface for balance and alignment, allowing seniors to perform exercises safely.

Enhanced Range of Motion: By utilizing the wall for certain movements, seniors can achieve a greater range of motion while maintaining proper form, contributing to improved flexibility.

Versatility: The wall adds versatility to exercises, allowing for modifications and creative variations to suit individual needs and goals.

5. Mind-Body Connection in Wall Pilates

Conscious Movement: Wall Pilates encourages a heightened awareness of movement, fostering a strong mind-body connection that enhances coordination and mental clarity.

Stress Reduction: Incorporating mindful breathing and intentional movement promotes relaxation, reducing stress levels and contributing to overall emotional well-being.

Understanding Wall Pilates lays the groundwork for a fulfilling and effective fitness practice. As you embark on your Wall Pilates journey, remember that it's not just about exercise; it's about cultivating a deeper connection with your body and embracing a holistic approach to senior well-being.

What is Pilates?

Pilates is a transformative and holistic approach to physical fitness that transcends conventional exercise routines. Developed by Joseph Pilates in the early 20th century, this method emphasizes the integration of mind and body, focusing on core strength, flexibility, and overall body awareness.

1. Holistic Fitness Philosophy

At its core, Pilates is not just a series of exercises; it's a philosophy that embraces the interconnectedness of physical and mental well-being. Joseph Pilates believed that a strong core, often referred to as the body's powerhouse, is the key to overall strength and stability. Pilates seeks to develop this core strength while considering the body as a whole, promoting balance and alignment.

2. Key Principles of Pilates

Centering: Pilates places a significant emphasis on the center of the body—the core muscles. All movements originate from the center, fostering stability and strength.

Control: Precise and controlled movements are the foundation of Pilates. Each exercise is performed with a focus on quality over quantity, promoting awareness and intention.

Breathing: Conscious and coordinated breathing is integrated into each movement. Proper breathing enhances oxygen flow, supports muscle engagement, and contributes to a sense of relaxation.

Precision: Pilates exercises are designed with attention to detail. Movements are executed with precision to target specific muscle groups, promoting efficiency and effectiveness.

Flow: Fluidity in transitions between exercises creates a seamless and connected workout experience. The emphasis on flow contributes to grace and ease in movement.

3. Versatility for All Fitness Levels
Pilates is a versatile fitness method that can be adapted to accommodate individuals of all fitness levels and ages. From beginners to advanced practitioners, Pilates offers a

range of exercises and modifications, making it accessible for everyone.

4. Equipment and Mat-Based Practices

Pilates can be practiced using specialized equipment, such as the reformer or Cadillac, which incorporate resistance to enhance the workout. Alternatively, mat-based Pilates utilizes body weight and minimal props, offering a convenient and accessible way to practice virtually anywhere.

5. Mind-Body Connection

One of the hallmark features of Pilates is the emphasis on the mind-body connection. Each movement is executed with awareness and intention, fostering a deep connection between physical actions and mental focus. This mindfulness not only enhances the effectiveness of the workout but also contributes to stress reduction and improved mental clarity.

6. Benefits Beyond the Physical
While Pilates is renowned for its physical benefits, including improved strength, flexibility, and posture, it also extends its positive impact to mental well-being. Regular practice is associated with reduced stress levels, enhanced concentration, and a heightened sense of overall wellness.

In essence, Pilates is a holistic journey that goes beyond the traditional notions of exercise. It's an invitation to cultivate strength, flexibility, and balance not just in the body, but in the mind and spirit as well.

Why Wall Pilates for Seniors?

Wall Pilates stands out as an ideal fitness modality for seniors, offering a unique blend of support, adaptability, and effectiveness. Tailored to address the specific needs of older adults, here are compelling reasons why Wall Pilates is a valuable addition to the well-being of seniors:

1. Gentle Support for Joint Health
Reduced Impact: The use of a wall provides gentle support, minimizing impact on joints. This is particularly beneficial for seniors, ensuring a low-impact workout that promotes joint health without compromising the effectiveness of the exercises.

Enhanced Stability: The wall acts as a stabilizing element, allowing seniors to perform exercises with increased stability. This is crucial for those with balance concerns, creating a safe environment for movement.

2. Adaptability to Individual Fitness Levels
Inclusive for All Ages: Wall Pilates is designed to be inclusive, accommodating seniors of all fitness levels and backgrounds. Whether you're a beginner or have been active throughout your life, the exercises can be tailored to suit your individual needs and capabilities.

Modifications for Specific Needs: Every exercise within Wall Pilates can be modified to address specific physical limitations or challenges, ensuring that seniors can engage in a personalized fitness routine that aligns with their unique requirements.

3. Focused Core Strength and Balance
Core Emphasis: Wall Pilates places a strong emphasis on core strength, targeting the muscles that support the spine and contribute to overall stability. This focus is particularly beneficial for seniors, as a strong core is essential for maintaining balance and preventing falls.

Balance Enhancement: Specific exercises within Wall Pilates are designed to enhance balance and stability, crucial elements for seniors seeking to maintain or improve their sense of equilibrium.

4. Mindful Movement and Cognitive Benefits

Mind-Body Connection: Wall Pilates encourages mindful movement, fostering a heightened awareness of the body and its capabilities. This mind-body connection not only enhances the effectiveness of the workout but also contributes to cognitive well-being.

Stress Reduction: The incorporation of breathing techniques and intentional movements in Wall Pilates promotes relaxation, reducing stress levels and supporting overall mental clarity. This holistic approach addresses both physical and mental aspects of well-being.

5. Accessible Anytime, Anywhere

Convenience: Wall Pilates can be practiced in the comfort of your home with minimal equipment, making it a convenient option for seniors. The adaptability of wall support allows for a versatile and accessible workout that can be integrated into daily routines.

No Age Limit: There's no age limit to the benefits of Wall Pilates. Whether you're looking to start a fitness routine later in life or continue an existing practice, Wall Pilates offers a welcoming and effective option for seniors.

6. Holistic Wellness Integration

Physical and Mental Well-Being: Wall Pilates goes beyond physical exercise, integrating mental and emotional well-being into the fitness experience. The support of the wall creates a holistic approach that nurtures overall wellness for seniors.

Long-Term Sustainability: The adaptability and gentle nature of Wall Pilates make it a sustainable long-term fitness option for seniors, promoting consistent engagement and contributing to a healthier and more active lifestyle.

Wall Pilates for seniors is a thoughtful and effective approach that combines support, adaptability, and holistic well-being. It's an invitation to embark on a fitness journey that is not only beneficial for the body but also enriching for the mind and spirit.

Setting Up Your Pilates Space

Creating a dedicated and comfortable Pilates space is essential for a fulfilling and effective workout experience. Whether you're a beginner or a seasoned practitioner, follow these steps to set up a Pilates space that inspires focus, motivation, and well-being.

1. Choosing the Right Space

Select a Quiet Area: Choose a space that is quiet and free from distractions. This will help you focus on your movements and maintain a mindful Pilates practice.

Sufficient Ventilation: Ensure good air circulation in the chosen space. Proper ventilation contributes to a comfortable and energizing workout environment.

2. Gathering Necessary Equipment
Pilates Mat: Invest in a high-quality Pilates or exercise mat to provide a comfortable and supportive surface for your workouts.

Resistance Bands: Depending on your routine, resistance bands can add an extra challenge to your exercises. They are versatile and great for strength training.

Pilates Ball: A small Pilates ball is excellent for targeting specific muscle groups, especially for core and stability exercises.

Pilates Ring: Also known as a magic circle, this is a great prop for toning and strengthening various muscle groups.

3. Positioning Your Mat and Props

Mat Placement: Lay your mat on a flat surface, ensuring it is level and free from any bumps or obstacles. The mat should provide enough space for your entire body during exercises.

Prop Accessibility: Arrange your resistance bands, Pilates ball, and Pilates ring within easy reach. This ensures a seamless flow during your workout without interruptions to fetch equipment.

4. Lighting and Ambiance

Natural Light: If possible, choose a space with natural light. Natural light not only enhances visibility but also contributes to a positive and energizing atmosphere.

Artificial Lighting: Install adjustable lighting to control the ambiance of your Pilates space. Soft and diffused lighting can create a calming environment.

5. Mirror Placement

Install a Mirror: Place a mirror in your Pilates space to monitor your form and alignment during exercises. A mirror is a valuable tool for ensuring proper technique and maximizing the benefits of each movement.

Full-Body View: Position the mirror so you can see your entire body, especially during exercises that involve complex movements or balance.

6. Music or Mindful Ambiance

Choose Inspirational Music: Create a playlist of calming or motivational music to enhance your Pilates experience. The right soundtrack can elevate your mood and keep you motivated.

Mindful Ambiance: Consider incorporating elements of mindfulness, such as soft instrumental music or nature sounds, to foster a sense of tranquility during your practice.

7. Personalization and Motivation

Add Personal Touches: Make your Pilates space inviting by adding personal touches such as plants, inspirational quotes, or artwork. Personalization can create a positive and motivating atmosphere.

Visual Goals: Display your fitness goals or a vision board in your Pilates space to serve as a visual reminder of your aspirations.

8. Safety Considerations
Clear Space: Ensure the area around your mat is clear of any obstacles to prevent accidents during exercises that involve movement or balance.

Secure Props: If using resistance bands or other props, ensure they are securely fastened to avoid any unexpected movements that could lead to injury.

By following these steps, you'll create a Pilates space that not only supports your physical practice but also nurtures a positive and motivating environment for your overall well-being.

Choosing the Right Wall

Selecting the appropriate wall for your Wall Pilates practice is a crucial step in ensuring a safe and effective workout. Here are key considerations to help you choose the right wall for your Wall Pilates sessions.

1. Sturdiness and Stability

Load-Bearing Wall: Opt for a load-bearing wall that can support your body weight and provide stability during exercises. Avoid walls with structural issues or instability.

Smooth Surface: Ensure the wall surface is smooth and free from any protrusions or irregularities that could impact your comfort or safety.

2. Adequate Space

Open Area: Choose a wall in a spacious and open area to allow for a full range of motion during exercises. Having ample space ensures you can perform movements without restrictions.

Clear Surroundings: Ensure the area around the wall is free from furniture or obstacles that could impede your movements or pose a safety risk.

3. Proximity to Your Pilates Space

Convenient Location: Ideally, the chosen wall should be in close proximity to your designated Pilates space. This ensures easy access and encourages regular practice.

Accessibility of Props: If you plan to use props or accessories during your Wall Pilates sessions, ensure they are easily accessible from your chosen wall.

4. Wall Height and Dimensions

Sufficient Height: The wall should have enough height to accommodate a variety of exercises. Consider your reach and the range of motion required for different movements.

Length and Width: While the length of the wall is essential, also consider the width. A wider wall allows for a variety of exercises, especially those involving lateral movements.

5. Wall Surface Material

Texture: Opt for a wall with a smooth surface to provide comfort during exercises that involve body contact with the wall. Avoid walls with overly textured surfaces that could cause discomfort.

Cleanability: If possible, choose a wall that is easy to clean. This ensures a hygienic practice space, especially if you plan to have regular contact with the wall during exercises.

6. Visual Appeal and Motivation
Aesthetics: While not a primary consideration, choosing a visually appealing wall can enhance your motivation and make your Pilates practice more enjoyable.

Natural Light: If possible, select a wall in an area with natural light. Natural light can positively impact your mood and create a more inviting atmosphere.

7. Safety Precautions

Wall Material Inspection: Before starting your Wall Pilates practice, inspect the chosen wall for any signs of damage or wear. Address any concerns to ensure a safe workout environment.

Flooring: Consider the type of flooring beneath the chosen wall. A padded or cushioned floor can provide additional comfort and safety during exercises.

By taking these considerations into account, you'll be able to choose a wall that enhances your Wall Pilates experience, providing the necessary support and stability for a rewarding and safe workout.

Necessary Equipment

Embarking on a Wall Pilates journey requires minimal equipment, carefully chosen to enhance the effectiveness of your exercises while maintaining simplicity and accessibility. Here's a breakdown of the necessary equipment for a fulfilling Wall Pilates practice.

1. Pilates Mat

Purpose: A high-quality Pilates or exercise mat provides a comfortable and supportive surface for your exercises, especially those that involve floor work or stretching.

Considerations: Choose a mat with adequate thickness to cushion your body during exercises, and ensure it has a non-slip surface to prevent any accidental slips.

2. Resistance Bands

Purpose: Resistance bands add an extra dimension to your Wall Pilates routine by providing resistance to your movements, targeting specific muscle groups and enhancing strength training.

Considerations: Opt for a set of varied resistance levels to accommodate different exercises and fitness levels. Make sure the bands are in good condition and free from any wear or tear.

3. Pilates Ball

Purpose: A small Pilates ball is an excellent prop for targeting specific muscle groups, especially those related to core strength and stability exercises against the wall.

Considerations: Choose a ball with an appropriate size for your body and fitness level. It should be firm enough to provide support but with a slight give for added comfort.

4. Pilates Ring (Magic Circle)
Purpose: The Pilates ring is a versatile prop that adds resistance and intensity to your Wall Pilates exercises, particularly those focused on toning and sculpting various muscle groups.

Considerations: Look for a Pilates ring with comfortable handles and sufficient resistance. Ensure that it's in good condition without any deformities.

5. Yoga Block (Optional)
Purpose: While not essential, a yoga block can be beneficial for modifying certain exercises or providing additional support during stretches.

Considerations: Choose a block made of dense foam for stability. Its primary purpose is to assist in achieving proper alignment and form.

6. Comfortable Workout Attire and Footwear
Purpose: Wearing comfortable and breathable workout attire allows for ease of movement during Wall Pilates exercises.

Considerations: Opt for clothing that doesn't restrict your movements and footwear with good grip, especially if you're performing standing exercises against the wall.

7. Water Bottle and Towel
Purpose: Staying hydrated during your Wall Pilates practice is essential. Having a water bottle and a towel on hand ensures you can maintain comfort and hydration throughout your workout.

Considerations: Choose a reusable water bottle and a small towel to keep you refreshed and dry during your session.

8. Mirror (Optional)

Purpose: While not equipment per se, having a mirror in your Pilates space can be advantageous for checking your form and alignment during exercises against the wall.

Considerations: Position the mirror in a way that allows you to see your entire body, especially during exercises that involve complex movements or balance.

By gathering these essential pieces of equipment, you'll be well-prepared for a dynamic and effective Wall Pilates practice. Keep in mind that simplicity and functionality are key as you create your ideal Wall Pilates workout environment.

Safety Considerations

Prioritizing safety is essential for a fulfilling and injury-free Wall Pilates practice. Whether you're a beginner or an experienced practitioner, adhere to these safety considerations to create a secure environment for your workouts.

1. Consultation with a Healthcare Professional

Health Assessment: Before starting any fitness program, including Wall Pilates, consult with a healthcare professional. They can assess your overall health and advise on any specific considerations or modifications needed based on your individual health profile.

Existing Conditions: Inform your healthcare provider of any existing medical conditions, injuries, or concerns that might impact your ability to engage in certain exercises.

2. Proper Warm-Up and Cool Down
Warm-Up: Begin each session with a thorough warm-up to prepare your muscles and joints for the exercises ahead. Incorporate dynamic movements to increase blood flow and flexibility.

Cool Down: Conclude your Wall Pilates session with a cool-down routine, including static stretches, to aid in muscle recovery and flexibility.

3. Appropriate Clothing and Footwear

Comfortable Attire: Wear comfortable and breathable workout attire that allows for a full range of motion. Avoid clothing that is too loose or restrictive.

Sturdy Footwear: If standing exercises are part of your routine, wear footwear with good grip to prevent slipping. Alternatively, practice barefoot if the surface is safe and comfortable.

4. Mindful Movements and Awareness
Conscious Execution: Perform each exercise with mindfulness and awareness of your body's movements. Avoid rushing through exercises and prioritize proper form over the number of repetitions.

Listen to Your Body: Pay attention to any discomfort, pain, or unusual sensations during exercises. If something doesn't feel right, stop the movement and reassess.

5. Adapt Exercises to Your Abilities

Modifications: Be willing to modify exercises based on your fitness level and any physical limitations. There's no one-size-fits-all approach, so adapt the routine to suit your abilities.

Progress Gradually: If you're new to Wall Pilates or returning after a break, progress gradually. Allow your body time to adapt and avoid pushing yourself too hard too soon.

6. Clear and Safe Practice Area

Clear Space: Ensure the area around your Pilates space is free from obstacles or tripping hazards. This is particularly important for exercises that involve movement or balance.

Secure Props: If using resistance bands or props, ensure they are securely fastened to prevent unexpected movements that could lead to injury.

7. Hydration and Rest

Stay Hydrated: Keep a water bottle nearby and stay hydrated throughout your workout. Dehydration can impact your performance and recovery.

Adequate Rest: Allow your body adequate rest between exercises and sessions.

Overtraining can lead to fatigue and increase the risk of injury.

8. Mirror Use for Form Checking (Optional)
Form Assessment: If using a mirror, periodically check your form and alignment to ensure you're maintaining proper posture during exercises.

Full-Body View: Position the mirror so you can see your entire body, especially during exercises that involve complex movements or balance.

By incorporating these safety considerations into your Wall Pilates practice, you'll create a secure and supportive environment that promotes both well-being and progress.

Basic Wall Pilates Exercises

These Wall Pilates exercises are designed to be gentle yet effective, catering to the unique needs of seniors. Incorporate these into your routine to enhance strength, flexibility, and balance while enjoying the support of the wall.

1. Wall Sit with Leg Lifts
Position: Stand with your back against the wall and lower into a seated position (as if sitting in an invisible chair).

Movement: Lift one leg at a time, extending it straight in front of you. Hold briefly and lower it back down. Repeat on the other leg.

Benefit: Strengthens the quadriceps, glutes, and improves balance.

2. Wall Push-Ups

Position: Face the wall, arms extended at shoulder height and palms on the wall.

Movement: Bend your elbows, bringing your chest toward the wall, and then push back to the starting position.

Benefit: Targets the chest, shoulders, and triceps, providing a modified push-up for upper body strength.

3. Wall Squats with Ball Squeeze

Position: Place a small Pilates ball between your knees. Stand with your back against the wall and feet hip-width apart.

Movement: Lower into a squat position while squeezing the ball between your knees. Hold briefly and return to the starting position.

Benefit: Strengthens the quads, hamstrings, and inner thighs while engaging the core.

4. Wall Roll-Downs
Position: Stand with your back against the wall, feet hip-width apart.

Movement: Slowly articulate your spine, rolling down towards the floor. Keep your knees slightly bent. Roll back up, one vertebra at a time.

Benefit: Improves spinal mobility and stretches the back and hamstrings.

5. Leg Press against the Wall
Position: Lie on your back with your feet against the wall, knees bent.

Movement: Press your feet into the wall, straightening your legs. Lower them back down without touching the floor.

Benefit: Targets the hamstrings, glutes, and thighs for lower body strength.

6. Wall Angel Stretch
Position: Stand with your back against the wall, arms at shoulder height.

Movement: Slide your arms up the wall, keeping them in contact with the wall, then slide them back down. Imagine drawing angel wings on the wall.

Benefit: Improves shoulder mobility and engages the upper back muscles.

7. Wall Calf Raises
Position: Stand facing the wall, with your hands resting lightly against it for support.

Movement: Lift your heels off the ground, rising onto the balls of your feet, then lower them back down.

Benefit: Strengthens the calf muscles and improves ankle stability.

Remember to perform these exercises at a pace that feels comfortable for you, and always prioritize proper form. If you have any existing health concerns, consult with your healthcare professional before starting a new exercise routine.

Warm-up Routine

A proper warm-up is essential for seniors to increase blood flow, loosen muscles, and enhance flexibility. These gentle and effective warm-up exercises will help prepare your body for a safe and enjoyable workout.

1. Neck Rolls

Movement: Slowly roll your head in a circular motion, first clockwise and then counterclockwise. Ensure gentle and controlled movements.

Benefit: Relieves tension in the neck and improves neck mobility.

2. Shoulder Rolls

Movement: Lift your shoulders towards your ears, then roll them back in a circular motion. Repeat in the opposite direction.

Benefit: Loosens up the shoulder muscles and promotes flexibility.

3. Arm Swings

Movement: Extend your arms to the sides and swing them back and forth gently. Gradually increase the range of motion.

Benefit: Warms up the shoulder joints and improves blood circulation.

4. Side Bends

Movement: Stand with feet shoulder-width apart. Gently lean from side to side, reaching one hand towards the knee while keeping the other arm overhead.

Benefit: Stretches the sides and promotes flexibility in the torso.

5. Hip Circles
Movement: Stand with feet hip-width apart. Circle your hips in a clockwise motion, then switch to counterclockwise.

Benefit: Warms up the hip joints and improves mobility.

6. Knee Lifts
Movement: While standing, lift one knee towards your chest, then lower it down. Repeat with the other knee.

Benefit: Warms up the hip flexors and improves balance.

7. Ankle Circles

Movement: Sit or stand with feet lifted slightly off the ground. Circle your ankles clockwise and then counterclockwise.

Benefit: Increases blood flow to the ankles and enhances ankle flexibility.

8. March in Place

Movement: Lift your knees high as you march in place. Swing your arms in a natural motion.

Benefit: Elevates the heart rate gradually and warms up major muscle groups.

9. Deep Breathing

Movement: Inhale deeply through your nose, expanding your chest and abdomen. Exhale slowly through your mouth.

Benefit: Promotes relaxation, focuses the mind, and prepares for mindful exercise.

Perform each of these exercises in a slow and controlled manner, and only go as far as feels comfortable for your body. The goal is to gently increase your heart rate and activate the major muscle groups.

Remember, if you experience pain or discomfort during the warm-up, stop the exercise and consult with your healthcare professional. This warm-up routine is

designed to set the stage for a safe and
enjoyable exercise session.

Gentle Stretching

Embrace the benefits of increased flexibility and improved range of motion with this gentle stretching routine designed for seniors. Perform these stretches at a comfortable pace, breathing deeply and mindfully. Remember to listen to your body and only stretch to the point of gentle tension, avoiding any pain.

1. Neck Stretch
Movement: Slowly tilt your head to one side, bringing your ear towards your shoulder. Hold for 15-20 seconds. Repeat on the other side.

Benefit: Relieves tension in the neck and shoulders.

2. Shoulder Stretch

Movement: Bring one arm across your chest and gently hold it with your opposite hand. Hold for 15-20 seconds. Repeat on the other arm.

Benefit: Stretches the shoulders and upper back.

3. Triceps Stretch

Movement: Raise one arm overhead and bend the elbow, reaching your hand down your back. Hold for 15-20 seconds. Repeat on the other arm.

Benefit: Targets the triceps and improves upper arm flexibility.

4. Wrist and Forearm Stretch

Movement: Extend one arm forward with the palm facing down. Use the opposite hand to gently press on the fingers. Hold for 15-20 seconds. Repeat on the other arm.

Benefit: Relieves tension in the wrists and forearms.

5. Seated Side Stretch

Movement: Sit comfortably with legs crossed. Reach one arm overhead and gently lean to the opposite side. Hold for 15-20 seconds. Repeat on the other side.

Benefit: Stretches the sides and promotes lateral flexibility.

6. Seated Forward Bend

Movement: Sit with legs extended in front. Hinge at the hips and reach towards your toes. Hold for 15-20 seconds.

Benefit: Stretches the hamstrings and lower back.

7. Hip Flexor Stretch
Movement: Stand with one foot forward and the other foot back. Gently lower your hips, feeling a stretch in the front of the hip of the back leg. Hold for 15-20 seconds. Repeat on the other side.

Benefit: Targets the hip flexors and improves hip mobility.

8. Calf Stretch

Movement: Stand facing a wall. Place one foot forward and the other foot back. Keep both heels on the ground and bend the front knee. Hold for 15-20 seconds. Repeat on the other side.

Benefit: Stretches the calves and promotes ankle flexibility.

9. Ankle Circles

Movement: Sit or stand with feet lifted slightly off the ground. Circle your ankles clockwise and then counterclockwise.

Benefit: Increases blood flow to the ankles and enhances ankle flexibility.

10. Deep Breathing and Gentle Twists

Movement: Sit or stand with a straight spine. Inhale deeply, and as you exhale, gently twist your upper body to one side. Hold for a few seconds and repeat on the other side.

Benefit: Enhances spinal flexibility and promotes relaxation.

Perform each stretch in a slow, controlled manner, and hold for 15-20 seconds. Remember to breathe deeply throughout each stretch. This routine can be done daily to maintain and improve flexibility while promoting overall well-being.

Breathing Techniques

Embrace the power of mindful breathing to promote relaxation, reduce stress, and enhance overall well-being. These gentle breathing exercises are tailored for seniors and can be incorporated into your daily routine.

1. Deep Belly Breathing (Diaphragmatic Breathing)

Technique:

Sit comfortably with your back straight or lie down.

Place one hand on your chest and the other on your abdomen.

Inhale slowly through your nose, allowing your abdomen to expand. Feel your hand on your abdomen rise.

Exhale slowly through your mouth, feeling your abdomen fall. Ensure your chest remains relatively still.

Benefit: Promotes relaxation, reduces anxiety, and increases oxygen flow to the body.

2. Box Breathing (Square Breathing)

Technique:

Inhale slowly through your nose for a count of four.

Hold your breath for a count of four.

Exhale slowly through your mouth for a count of four.

Pause and hold your breath for another count of four.

Benefit: Calms the nervous system, improves focus, and reduces stress.

3. Alternate Nostril Breathing (Nadi Shodhana)

Technique:

Sit comfortably with a straight spine.

Use your right thumb to close your right nostril and inhale through your left nostril.

Close your left nostril with your right ring finger, release your right nostril, and exhale.

Inhale through your right nostril, close it, release your left nostril, and exhale. This completes one cycle.

Benefit: Balances energy, reduces stress, and enhances mental clarity.

4. Pursed-Lip Breathing

Technique:
Inhale slowly through your nose for a count of two.
Pucker your lips as if preparing to blow out a candle.
Exhale slowly and gently through pursed lips for a count of four.
Benefit: Improves lung function, reduces shortness of breath, and promotes relaxation.

5. 4-7-8 Breathing

Technique:
Inhale quietly through your nose for a count of four.

Hold your breath for a count of seven.

Exhale completely through your mouth for a count of eight.

Benefit: Induces relaxation, reduces stress, and promotes a sense of calm.

6. Mindful Breath Awareness

Technique:

Sit comfortably and close your eyes.

Focus your attention on your breath.

Notice the sensation of each inhale and exhale.

If your mind wanders, gently bring it back to your breath.

Benefit: Enhances mindfulness, reduces anxiety, and promotes a sense of presence.

Incorporate these breathing techniques into your daily routine, dedicating a few minutes to mindful breathing. These exercises can be done seated or lying down, making them accessible and adaptable to your preferences.

Intermediate Wall Pilates Exercises

Take your Wall Pilates practice to the next level with these intermediate exercises designed specifically for seniors. As you progress, remember to maintain proper form, breathe deeply, and listen to your body. Consult with your healthcare professional before attempting new exercises, and modify as needed to suit your individual needs.

1. Wall Squats with Ball Squeeze and Leg Lifts

Position: Place a small Pilates ball between your knees. Stand with your back against the wall and lower into a squat position.

Movement:

Hold the squat position with the ball squeezed.

Lift one leg at a time, extending it straight in front of you.

Benefit: Targets the quadriceps, hamstrings, and improves balance.

2. Wall Plank with Leg Lifts

Position: Face the wall and place your hands on the wall at shoulder height. Walk your feet back, forming a plank position.

Movement:

Lift one leg at a time, engaging your core to maintain a straight body.

Hold each leg lift for a few seconds before alternating.

Benefit: Strengthens the core, shoulders, and improves overall body awareness.

3. Wall Push-Ups with Knee Tucks
Position: Face the wall with hands at shoulder height. Perform a push-up against the wall.

Movement:
After each push-up, bring one knee towards your chest, engaging the abdominal muscles.
Alternate between knees with each push-up.
Benefit: Targets the chest, shoulders, and engages the core.

4. Wall Bridge with Marching
Position: Lie on your back with feet against the wall and knees bent.

Movement:

Lift your hips towards the ceiling to form a bridge.

While in the bridge position, march your knees, lifting one foot at a time.

Benefit: Strengthens the glutes, hamstrings, and improves hip stability.

5. Side Plank with Leg Lifts

Position: Stand facing the wall and place one forearm on the wall at shoulder height.

Step your feet back, forming a side plank.

Movement:

Lift the top leg towards the ceiling.

Hold for a few seconds before lowering and repeating on the other side.

Benefit: Targets the obliques, hips, and improves lateral stability.

6. Wall Roll-Ups

Position: Sit with your back against the wall and legs extended.

Movement:

Slowly roll down to lie on your back.

Roll back up, engaging your core and maintaining control.

Benefit: Improves abdominal strength and spinal mobility.

7. Wall Squat with Overhead Reach

Position: Stand with your back against the wall and lower into a squat position.

Movement:

As you lower into the squat, reach both arms overhead.

Hold the squat position with overhead arms.

Benefit: Engages the entire lower body and improves shoulder flexibility.

8. Wall Teaser

Position: Sit with your back against the wall and legs lifted, forming a V shape.

Movement:

Slowly lower your upper body towards the floor while extending your legs.

Return to the starting V shape.

Benefit: Challenges core strength and improves overall body control.

9. Wall Lunge with Twist

Position: Stand facing the wall and take a step back with one foot, forming a lunge position.

Movement:

Rotate your torso towards the front leg.

Return to the starting position and repeat on the other side.

Benefit: Strengthens the legs, improves hip mobility, and engages the core.

10. Wall Pike Stretch

Position: Stand facing the wall and place your hands on the wall at shoulder height.

Movement:

Hinge at the hips, bringing your torso towards the wall.

Hold the pike stretch, feeling the stretch in your hamstrings and lower back.

Benefit: Stretches the hamstrings and promotes spinal flexibility.

Incorporate these intermediate Wall Pilates exercises into your routine gradually, focusing on proper form and controlled movements. As always, listen to your body and modify exercises as needed. If you have any concerns or medical conditions, consult with your healthcare professional before attempting new exercises.

Core Strengthening

A strong core is the foundation for stability and mobility, crucial aspects of maintaining an active and independent lifestyle. These core strengthening exercises are designed for seniors, focusing on building strength in the abdominal, back, and hip muscles. Always consult with your healthcare professional before starting a new exercise routine and ensure that you listen to your body throughout the exercises.

1. Seated Leg Lifts

Position: Sit on a stable chair with your back straight and feet flat on the floor.

Movement:

Lift one leg straight out in front of you, engaging your abdominal muscles.

Lower the leg back down and repeat on the other side.

Benefit: Targets the lower abdominal muscles and improves hip flexibility.

2. Pelvic Tilts

Position: Lie on your back with knees bent and feet flat on the floor.

Movement:

Inhale to prepare, exhale and gently tilt your pelvis up towards the ceiling.

Inhale to return to the starting position.

Benefit: Strengthens the lower back and improves pelvic stability.

3. Standing Oblique Crunches

Position: Stand with feet hip-width apart and hands placed behind your head.

Movement:

Lift one knee towards your elbow on the same side, engaging your obliques.

Return to the starting position and repeat on the other side.

Benefit: Targets the oblique muscles and improves balance.

4. Chair Plank

Position: Sit on the edge of a sturdy chair with your hands placed on the seat, fingers pointing forward.

Movement:

Walk your feet forward until your body forms a straight line.

Hold the plank position, engaging your core muscles.

Benefit: Strengthens the entire core, including the abdominal and back muscles.

5. Knee-to-Chest Stretch

Position: Lie on your back with knees bent and feet flat on the floor.

Movement:

Bring one knee towards your chest, holding it with both hands.

Hold for a few seconds and switch to the other leg.

Benefit: Stretches the lower back and hip flexors while engaging the core.

6. Seated Russian Twists

Position: Sit on the floor with knees bent and feet flat on the ground. Lean back slightly, keeping your back straight.

Movement:

Twist your torso to one side, bringing your hands towards the floor.

Return to the center and twist to the other side.

Benefit: Targets the obliques and improves spinal mobility.

7. Leg Raises

Position: Lie on your back with legs extended.

Movement:

Lift both legs towards the ceiling, engaging your abdominal muscles.

Lower your legs back down without touching the floor.

Benefit: Strengthens the lower abdominal muscles and improves hip flexibility.

8. Side Plank with Knee Lift

Position: Start in a side plank position on your elbow.

Movement:

Lift your top leg towards the ceiling while keeping your body in a straight line.

Lower the leg back down and switch to the other side.

Benefit: Targets the obliques and improves lateral stability.

9. Bird-Dog Exercise

Position: Start on hands and knees in a tabletop position.

Movement:

Extend one arm forward while lifting the opposite leg straight back.

Hold for a few seconds, then switch sides.

Benefit: Engages the core muscles and improves balance.

10. Standing March

Position: Stand with feet hip-width apart.

Movement:

Lift one knee towards your chest while swinging the opposite arm forward.

Alternate between legs in a marching motion.

Benefit: Engages the core and improves balance and coordination.

Incorporate these core strengthening exercises into your routine to enhance stability, support your spine, and improve overall functional strength. Start with a few repetitions and gradually increase as you feel comfortable. Always prioritize proper form and consult with your healthcare professional if you have any concerns.

Balance and Stability

Improving balance and stability is essential for maintaining independence and preventing falls, especially as we age. These exercises are designed specifically for seniors to enhance proprioception, strengthen stabilizing muscles, and promote confidence in daily activities. Always consult with your healthcare professional before starting a new exercise routine, and perform these exercises in a safe and supportive environment.

1. Heel-to-Toe Walk

Setup: Stand with your heel of one foot touching the toes of the other foot.

Movement:

Take a step forward, placing the heel of the front foot directly in front of the toes of the back foot.

Repeat, walking in a straight line.

Benefit: Improves balance and encourages a heel-to-toe weight shift.

2. Single Leg Stance

Setup: Stand near a sturdy chair or counter for support.

Movement:

Lift one foot off the ground, balancing on the opposite leg.

Hold the position for as long as comfortable, aiming for 10-30 seconds.

Switch to the other leg.

Benefit: Strengthens stabilizing muscles in the legs and improves overall balance.

3. Toe Taps

Setup: Stand with feet hip-width apart.

Movement:

Lift one foot and tap the toes on the ground in front of you.

Return the foot to the starting position.

Repeat on the other leg.

Benefit: Enhances balance and focuses on controlled weight shifts.

4. Side Leg Lifts

Setup: Stand near a supportive surface.

Movement:

Lift one leg out to the side, keeping it straight.

Hold for a moment, then lower the leg back down.

Repeat on the other leg.

Benefit: Targets the hip abductors and improves lateral stability.

5. Tandem Stance

Setup: Stand with one foot in front of the other, heel to toe.

Movement:

Hold the tandem stance, balancing on the front foot.

Switch the position of your feet and repeat.

Benefit: Challenges balance and coordination by narrowing your base of support.

6. Chair Squats

Setup: Stand with feet hip-width apart, facing a sturdy chair.

Movement:

Lower into a squat, reaching back towards the chair with your hips.

Stand back up, engaging your leg and core muscles.

Benefit: Strengthens the lower body and promotes controlled movements.

7. Clock Reach

Setup: Imagine standing in the center of a clock face.

Movement:

Lift one leg and reach it forward to 12 o'clock.

Return to the center and reach the leg to 3 o'clock, then 6 o'clock, and 9 o'clock.

Repeat on the other leg.

Benefit: Improves dynamic balance and stability in different directions.

8. Standing Calf Raises

Setup: Stand near a wall or counter for support.

Movement:

Lift both heels off the ground, rising onto the balls of your feet.

Lower your heels back down.

Benefit: Strengthens the calf muscles and improves ankle stability.

9. Marching in Place with Arm Swings

Movement:

Stand with feet hip-width apart.

Lift your knees towards your chest in a marching motion.

Swing your arms in a controlled and rhythmic manner.

Benefit: Enhances balance and coordination in a dynamic way.

10. Weight Shifts

Setup: Stand with feet hip-width apart.

Movement:

Shift your weight onto one leg, lifting the opposite foot slightly.

Return to center and shift your weight to the other leg.

Benefit: Improves weight distribution and challenges lateral stability.

Perform these exercises regularly, aiming for a well-rounded balance routine. Start with a few repetitions and gradually increase as you feel more confident. If needed, have a stable surface nearby for support. Consistency is key in building and maintaining balance and stability.

Flexibility Training

Flexibility is a key component of overall fitness, promoting joint health, reducing the risk of injury, and improving range of motion. These gentle and effective flexibility exercises are designed specifically for seniors. Always consult with your healthcare professional before starting a new exercise routine and perform these exercises in a controlled and comfortable environment.

1. Neck Stretch

Movement:
Slowly tilt your head to one side, bringing your ear towards your shoulder.
Hold for 15-30 seconds.
Repeat on the other side.

Benefit: Relieves tension in the neck and promotes neck flexibility.

2. Shoulder Rolls

Movement:
Lift your shoulders towards your ears, then roll them back in a circular motion.
Repeat in the opposite direction.
Benefit: Loosens up the shoulder muscles and promotes flexibility.

3. Arm and Chest Opener

Movement:
Clasp your hands behind your back.
Straighten your arms and lift them slightly, opening your chest.

Benefit: Stretches the chest, shoulders, and improves posture.

4. Wrist and Forearm Stretch

Movement:

Extend one arm forward with the palm facing down.

Use the opposite hand to gently press on the fingers.

Hold for 15-30 seconds.

Repeat on the other arm.

Benefit: Relieves tension in the wrists and forearms.

5. Side Bends

Movement:

Stand with feet shoulder-width apart.

Gently lean from side to side, reaching one hand towards the knee while keeping the other arm overhead.

Benefit: Stretches the sides and promotes lateral flexibility.

6. Seated Forward Bend

Movement:

Sit with legs extended in front.

Hinge at the hips and reach towards your toes.

Benefit: Stretches the hamstrings and lower back.

7. Hip Flexor Stretch

Movement:

Kneel on one knee with the other foot in front, forming a lunge.

Gently press your hips forward, feeling a stretch in the hip of the back leg.

Benefit: Targets the hip flexors and improves hip mobility.

8. Seated Leg Cross Stretch

Movement:

Sit with legs crossed.

Gently twist your torso towards one side, using the opposite arm for support.

Benefit: Stretches the spine and promotes rotational flexibility.

9. Ankle Circles

Movement:

Sit or stand with feet lifted slightly off the ground.

Circle your ankles clockwise and then counterclockwise.

Benefit: Increases blood flow to the ankles and enhances ankle flexibility.

10. Deep Breathing and Gentle Twists

Movement:

Sit or stand with a straight spine.

Inhale deeply, and as you exhale, gently twist your upper body to one side.

Hold for a few seconds and repeat on the other side.

Benefit: Enhances spinal flexibility and promotes relaxation.

Perform these flexibility exercises regularly, aiming for a well-rounded routine. Hold each stretch for 15-30 seconds, breathing deeply and avoiding any pain. Focus on the sensations in your muscles and joints, and gradually increase the intensity of the stretches over time.

Advanced Wall Pilates Techniques

Take your Wall Pilates practice to the next level with these advanced techniques designed to challenge and elevate your strength, stability, and flexibility. Ensure you have a solid foundation in basic and intermediate Wall Pilates exercises before attempting these advanced techniques. Always consult with your healthcare professional before starting a new exercise routine and perform these exercises in a controlled and safe environment.

1. Wall Plank with Knee Tucks and Leg Extensions

Position: Face the wall and place your hands on the wall at shoulder height. Walk your feet back, forming a plank position.

Movement:

Bring one knee towards your chest in a tuck.

Extend the same leg straight back, engaging the glutes.

Repeat on the other leg.

Benefit: Targets the core, shoulders, and improves overall body control.

2. Wall Pike with Single Leg Lifts

Position: Assume a plank position facing the wall with hands at shoulder height.

Movement:

Lift one leg towards the ceiling in a pike position.

Hold for a moment before lowering the leg back down.

Repeat on the other leg.

Benefit: Strengthens the core, shoulders, and challenges balance.

3. Wall L-Sit

Position: Sit on the floor with your back against the wall and legs extended.

Movement:

Lift both legs off the ground, forming an L-shape with your body.

Hold the L-sit position for as long as comfortable.

Benefit: Engages the core, hip flexors, and improves overall body strength.

4. Wall Push-Ups with Mountain Climbers

Position: Face the wall with hands at shoulder height. Perform a push-up against the wall.

Movement:

After each push-up, bring one knee towards your chest in a mountain climber motion. Alternate between knees with each push-up. Benefit: Targets the chest, shoulders, and adds a dynamic element to the exercise.

5. Wall Scissor Kicks

Position: Lie on your back with legs extended, pressing against the wall.

Movement:

Lift both legs towards the ceiling.

Lower one leg towards the floor while keeping the other leg lifted.

Switch legs in a scissor-like motion.

Benefit: Strengthens the core, hip flexors, and improves lower abdominal strength.

6. Wall Teaser with Twist

Position: Sit with your back against the wall and legs lifted, forming a V shape.

Movement:

Lower your upper body towards the floor while twisting to one side.

Return to the starting V shape and twist to the other side.

Benefit: Challenges core strength and adds a rotational element to the exercise.

7. Wall Side Plank with Hip Dips

Position: Start in a side plank position facing the wall on your forearm.

Movement:

Dip your hips towards the floor.

Lift your hips back up to the side plank position.

Benefit: Targets the obliques and improves lateral stability.

8. Wall Roll-Up to V-Sit

Position: Sit on the floor with your back against the wall and legs extended.

Movement:

Slowly roll down to lie on your back.

Roll back up, lifting your legs and upper body simultaneously into a V-sit position.

Benefit: Engages the entire core and challenges overall body coordination.

9. Wall Plank with Leg Circles

Position: Face the wall and place your hands on the wall at shoulder height. Walk your feet back, forming a plank position.

Movement:

Lift one leg towards the ceiling and draw small circles with your foot.

Reverse the direction of the circles.

Benefit: Engages the core, shoulders, and improves hip mobility.

10. Wall Reverse Plank with Leg Lifts

Position: Sit with your hands behind you on the floor and legs extended against the wall.

Movement:

Lift your hips towards the ceiling into a reverse plank position.

Lift one leg towards the ceiling and hold for a moment before lowering.

Benefit: Targets the core, glutes, and improves overall body strength.

Incorporate these advanced Wall Pilates techniques into your routine gradually, focusing on proper form and controlled movements. As always, listen to your body and modify exercises as needed. If you have any concerns or medical conditions, consult with your healthcare professional before attempting new exercises.

Building Strength

Strength training is a key component of a well-rounded fitness routine, offering numerous benefits for seniors, including increased muscle mass, improved bone density, and enhanced functional abilities. These strength-building exercises are designed to be safe, effective, and adaptable to various fitness levels. Always consult with your healthcare professional before starting a new exercise routine and perform these exercises in a controlled and safe environment.

1. Bodyweight Squats
Movement:
Stand with feet hip-width apart.

Lower your body as if sitting back into a chair.

Keep your chest up, and knees aligned with your toes.

Return to the starting position.

Benefit: Strengthens the lower body, including the quadriceps and glutes.

2. Wall Push-Ups

Movement:

Stand facing a wall with hands at shoulder height.

Perform a push-up by leaning towards the wall.

Push back to the starting position.

Benefit: Targets the chest, shoulders, and triceps.

3. Chair Squats

Movement:

Stand with feet hip-width apart, facing away from a sturdy chair.

Lower your body towards the chair, then stand back up.

Benefit: Strengthens the lower body and promotes controlled movements.

4. Leg Press Against the Wall

Movement:

Sit with your back against the wall and knees bent.

Press your feet into the wall, straightening your legs.

Lower back down to the starting position.

Benefit: Targets the quadriceps and hamstrings.

5. Seated Leg Raises

Movement:

Sit on a stable chair with your back straight.

Lift one leg straight out in front of you.

Lower the leg back down and repeat on the other side.

Benefit: Strengthens the quadriceps and improves hip flexibility.

6. Resistance Band Rows

Movement:

Sit or stand with a resistance band anchored at chest height.

Hold the ends of the band and pull your elbows back.

Squeeze your shoulder blades together and return to the starting position.

Benefit: Targets the upper back muscles.

7. Bicep Curls with Light Weights

Movement:

Stand with a weight in each hand, arms extended.

Bend your elbows and lift the weights towards your shoulders.

Lower the weights back down.

Benefit: Strengthens the biceps.

8. Chair Dips

Movement:

Sit on the edge of a sturdy chair with hands gripping the edges.

Slide your hips off the chair and lower your body.

Push back up to the starting position.

Benefit: Targets the triceps and shoulders.

9. Standing Calf Raises

Movement:

Stand with feet hip-width apart.

Lift your heels off the ground, rising onto the balls of your feet.

Lower your heels back down.

Benefit: Strengthens the calf muscles and improves ankle stability.

10. Plank

Movement:

Start on hands and knees in a tabletop position.

Extend your legs straight behind you, forming a plank position.

Hold the plank, engaging your core muscles.

Benefit: Targets the core, shoulders, and improves overall body stability.

Perform these strength-building exercises 2-3 times per week, allowing for a day of rest between sessions. Start with a few repetitions and gradually increase as you feel more comfortable. Focus on proper form, breathing deeply, and listen to your body. If needed, have a stable surface nearby for support.

Coordination Exercises

Improving coordination is essential for maintaining independence and overall well-being as we age. These exercises focus on enhancing motor skills, balance, and cognitive function. Always consult with your healthcare professional before starting a new exercise routine and perform these exercises in a controlled and safe environment.

1. Marching in Place with Arm Movements

Movement:
Stand with feet hip-width apart.
Lift your knees towards your chest in a marching motion.

Add arm movements, swinging them in a controlled and rhythmic manner.

Benefit: Enhances balance and coordination in a dynamic way.

2. Balloon Toss

Equipment:

Balloons (light and easy to catch).

Activity:

Stand with a partner or against a wall.

Toss the balloon back and forth, aiming for controlled catches.

Benefit: Improves hand-eye coordination and reaction time.

3. Figure 8 Walking

Setup:

Place two objects on the ground in the shape of a figure 8.

Movement:

Walk around the objects, following the figure 8 pattern.

Benefit: Challenges balance and coordination while walking.

4. Cone Drill

Equipment:

Cones or markers.

Activity:

Set up a series of cones in a pattern on the ground.

Navigate through the cones following the pattern.

Benefit: Enhances agility, spatial awareness, and coordination.

5. Tap and Touch

Movement:

Stand with feet hip-width apart.

Tap one foot to the side and touch the floor with the opposite hand.

Return to the starting position and switch sides.

Benefit: Improves coordination between limbs and enhances lateral movement.

6. Cross-Crawl Exercise

Movement:

Stand with feet hip-width apart.

Lift one knee towards your chest while bringing the opposite elbow towards the knee.

Repeat on the other side.

Benefit: Stimulates both sides of the brain and improves coordination.

7. Ladder Drills

Equipment:

Agility ladder.

Activity:

Perform various footwork patterns through the ladder.

Benefit: Enhances foot speed, agility, and overall coordination.

8. Tai Chi

Movement:
Engage in slow, deliberate movements, focusing on balance and coordination.
Benefit: Improves coordination, flexibility, and mindfulness.

9. Reaction Ball Bounces

Equipment:
Reaction ball (bounces unpredictably).

Activity:

Bounce the reaction ball against a wall and catch it as it rebounds in unpredictable directions.

Benefit: Challenges reaction time and hand-eye coordination.

10. Seated Marching with Arm Crosses

Movement:

Sit on a stable chair.

Lift your knees in a marching motion while crossing your arms over your chest.

Benefit: Improves coordination between upper and lower body.

Incorporate these coordination exercises into your routine regularly. Start with a few minutes each day and gradually increase the duration as you feel more comfortable. Focus on the quality of movement, and have fun challenging your coordination skills.

Modifications for Individual Needs

Adapting exercises to meet individual needs ensures a safe and enjoyable fitness experience. Whether dealing with mobility issues, joint concerns, or other health conditions, these modifications can help tailor exercises to specific requirements. Always consult with your healthcare professional before starting a new exercise routine and make adjustments based on personal comfort and capability.

1. Chair Support

Modification:
Incorporate a stable chair for support during standing exercises.

Use the chair as a prop for balance during activities like leg lifts or squats.

Benefit:

Provides stability for those with balance or mobility concerns.

Enables participation in standing exercises with added support.

2. Reduced Range of Motion

Modification:

Perform exercises with a smaller range of motion.

For example, during squats, only lower partway rather than going into a full squat.

Benefit:

Reduces joint strain for individuals with limited flexibility or joint issues.

Allows participation in exercises with a controlled range of motion.

3. Seated Options

Modification:

Choose seated variations of exercises.

For instance, perform seated leg lifts or seated marches.

Benefit:

Ideal for individuals with limited mobility or those who prefer a seated position.

Reduces stress on the joints while still engaging muscles.

4. Lighter Resistance

Modification:
Use lighter weights or resistance bands.
Decrease the intensity to a level that feels comfortable.

Benefit:
Suitable for individuals with joint issues or those new to strength training.
Allows gradual progression without straining muscles.

5. Gentle Stretching

Modification:
Focus on gentle stretching exercises.
Perform stretches with a comfortable and controlled effort.

Benefit:

Ideal for individuals with stiffness or joint concerns.

Promotes flexibility without causing discomfort.

6. Slow Paced Movements

Modification:

Perform exercises at a slower pace.

Emphasize controlled and deliberate movements.

Benefit:

Reduces the risk of injury by allowing individuals to maintain better control.

Suitable for those who prefer a slower and more mindful approach.

7. Breathing Focus

Modification:
Place emphasis on controlled breathing during exercises.
Inhale and exhale consciously, promoting relaxation.

Benefit:
Helps manage stress and anxiety during physical activity.
Improves focus and enhances overall well-being.

8. Water Exercises

Modification:
Engage in water-based exercises.

Water provides buoyancy and reduces impact on joints.

Benefit:

Ideal for individuals with arthritis or joint pain.

Offers a supportive environment for cardiovascular and strength exercises.

9. Frequent Breaks

Modification:

Take breaks as needed.

Listen to your body and rest when required.

Benefit:

Prevents overexertion and fatigue.

Allows individuals to pace themselves according to their energy levels.

10. Personalized Routine

Modification:

Tailor a routine based on individual preferences and limitations.

Choose exercises that align with personal goals and health conditions.

Benefit:

Ensures a customized and enjoyable fitness experience.

Addresses specific needs and promotes long-term adherence.

Always prioritize safety and comfort when modifying exercises. Regularly reassess individual needs and make adjustments accordingly. A personalized approach to fitness fosters a positive and sustainable exercise routine.

Incorporating Props

Using props can enhance the effectiveness and enjoyment of your exercise routine. These versatile tools add variety, challenge different muscle groups, and promote functional movements. Always consult with your healthcare professional before incorporating new props into your fitness regimen. Here are some senior-friendly exercises with props:

1. Resistance Bands

Exercise: Seated Leg Press

- Sit on a stable chair.
- Place a resistance band around the balls of your feet.
- Press your legs forward against the resistance of the band.

Benefit: Strengthens the quadriceps and hamstrings.

2. Light Dumbbells or Water Bottles

Exercise: Shoulder Press

- Sit or stand with a weight in each hand.
- Lift the weights from shoulder height to overhead.
- Lower the weights back down.

Benefit: Strengthens the shoulder muscles and improves arm strength.

3. Balance Discs or Stability Cushions

Exercise: Seated Balance

- Sit on a stability cushion or balance disc.
- Practice maintaining balance while engaging your core.

Benefit: Improves core stability and balance.

4. Soft Medicine Ball

Exercise: Seated Medicine Ball Twist

- Sit on a stable chair with a soft medicine ball.
- Hold the ball with both hands and twist your torso side to side.

Benefit: Targets the obliques and improves rotational flexibility.

5. Pilates Ring (Magic Circle)

Exercise: Inner Thigh Squeeze

- Place the Pilates ring between your thighs while seated.
- Squeeze the ring by engaging your inner thigh muscles.

Benefit: Strengthens the inner thighs and pelvic floor muscles.

6. Foam Roller

Exercise: Seated Leg Massage

- Sit on a stable chair with a foam roller under one foot.
- Roll the foot over the foam roller, massaging the sole.

Benefit: Promotes foot flexibility and relieves tension.

7. Yoga Blocks

Exercise: Seated Hip Opener

- Sit on the floor with yoga blocks under your knees.
- Allow your knees to open outward, stretching the hips.

Benefit: Improves hip flexibility and mobility.

8. Balance Ball

Exercise: Wall Squats with Ball

- Place a stability ball between your back and a wall.
- Lower into a squat position while keeping the ball against the wall.

Benefit: Strengthens the quadriceps, glutes, and improves posture.

9. Stretching Strap or Towel

Exercise: Seated Hamstring Stretch

- Sit with legs extended.
- Place a stretching strap or towel around one foot and gently lean forward.

Benefit: Promotes hamstring flexibility and lower back release.

10. Ankle Weights

Exercise: Seated Leg Raises with Ankle Weights

- Sit on a stable chair with ankle weights on your legs.
- Lift one leg at a time in a controlled manner.

Benefit: Strengthens the hip flexors and quadriceps.

When incorporating props, start with low resistance or intensity and gradually progress. Ensure proper form and technique to prevent injury. Listen to your body and choose props that suit your fitness level and goals. Props can add an exciting dimension to your workouts while catering to your individual needs.

Using Resistance Bands

Resistance bands are excellent for building strength, improving flexibility, and enhancing overall fitness. These exercises are designed to be senior-friendly, focusing on functionality and joint health. Always consult with your healthcare professional before starting a new exercise routine and ensure that the resistance level of the bands is appropriate for your fitness level.

1. Seated Leg Press

Setup:
Sit on a stable chair with your back straight. Loop the resistance band around the balls of your feet.

Movement:

Press your legs forward against the resistance of the band.

Slowly return to the starting position.

Benefit:

Strengthens the quadriceps and hamstrings.

Improves lower body strength and endurance.

2. Seated Row

Setup:

Sit on a stable chair with legs extended and the band securely anchored.

Hold the band with both hands, arms extended in front.

Movement:

Pull the band towards your chest, squeezing your shoulder blades.

Slowly release back to the starting position.

Benefit:

Targets the muscles of the upper back.

Improves posture and upper body strength.

3. Bicep Curl

Setup:

Sit or stand with the resistance band under the arches of your feet.

Hold the ends of the band with palms facing forward.

Movement:

Curl the hands towards your shoulders, engaging the biceps.

Slowly lower the hands back down.

Benefit:

Strengthens the biceps and forearms.

Enhances arm muscle tone and functionality.

4. Leg Abduction

Setup:

Secure one end of the resistance band to a stable anchor.

Attach the other end to your ankle.

Movement:

Lift the leg to the side against the resistance of the band.

Return the leg to the starting position.

Benefit:

Targets the hip abductors and outer thigh muscles.

Improves hip stability and strength.

5. Lateral Shoulder Raise

Setup:

Stand on the middle of the resistance band with feet shoulder-width apart.

Hold the ends of the band with palms facing your thighs.

Movement:

Lift your arms to the sides, keeping a slight bend in the elbows.

Lower the arms back down.

Benefit:

Targets the lateral deltoids (shoulder muscles).

Enhances shoulder strength and stability.

6. Seated Lat Pulldown

Setup:

Sit on a stable chair with the band securely anchored overhead.

Hold the ends of the band with palms facing forward.

Movement:

Pull the band down towards your chest, engaging the lat muscles.

Slowly release back to the starting position.

Benefit:

Targets the latissimus dorsi (back muscles).

Improves upper body strength and posture.

7. Clamshell

Setup:

Place a resistance band just above your knees.

Lie on your side with knees bent and ankles stacked.

Movement:

Lift the top knee towards the ceiling against the resistance of the band.

Lower the knee back down.

Benefit:
Activates the hip abductors and gluteus medius.
Enhances hip stability and strengthens the glutes.

8. Tricep Extension
Setup:
Sit or stand with the resistance band anchored behind you.
Hold one end of the band with your hand overhead.

Movement:
Extend your arm overhead, engaging the triceps.

Slowly bend the elbow to return to the starting position.

Benefit:

Targets the triceps (back of the arms).

Improves arm strength and tone.

When using resistance bands, focus on controlled movements, proper form, and breathing. Start with a light resistance and gradually progress as your strength improves. The versatility of resistance bands makes them an excellent addition to any senior fitness routine.

Small Props for Added Challenge

Incorporating small props into your workouts not only adds a fun element but also provides an extra challenge for various muscle groups. These exercises focus on functional movements and improving overall strength and balance. Always consult with your healthcare professional before introducing new props into your fitness routine. Here are some senior-friendly exercises with small props:

1. Soft Medicine Ball

Exercise: Seated Medicine Ball Twist

- Sit on a stable chair with a soft medicine ball.
- Hold the ball with both hands and twist your torso side to side.

Benefit:

Targets the obliques and improves rotational flexibility.

2. Pilates Ring (Magic Circle)

Exercise: Inner Thigh Squeeze

- Place the Pilates ring between your thighs while seated.
- Squeeze the ring by engaging your inner thigh muscles.

Benefit:

Strengthens the inner thighs and pelvic floor muscles.

3. Foam Roller

Exercise: Seated Leg Massage

- Sit on a stable chair with a foam roller under one foot.

- Roll the foot over the foam roller, massaging the sole.

Benefit:

Promotes foot flexibility and relieves tension.

4. Yoga Blocks

Exercise: Seated Hip Opener

- Sit on the floor with yoga blocks under your knees.
- Allow your knees to open outward, stretching the hips.

Benefit:

Improves hip flexibility and mobility.

5. Balance Cushion

Exercise: Standing Balance Challenge

- Stand on a balance cushion with feet hip-width apart.

- Hold onto a stable surface for support if needed.

Benefit:

Enhances balance and stability.

Engages core muscles for added strength.

6. Hand Weights (Dumbbells or Water Bottles)

Exercise: Dynamic Arm Circles

- Hold a lightweight in each hand (dumbbells or water bottles).
- Extend your arms to the sides and perform small circles.

Benefit:

Tones shoulder muscles.

Adds resistance for improved arm strength.

7. Ankle Weights

Exercise: Seated Leg Raises with Ankle Weights

- Sit on a stable chair with ankle weights on your legs.
- Lift one leg at a time in a controlled manner.

Benefit:

Strengthens the hip flexors and quadriceps.

8. Resistance Bands with Handles

Exercise: Standing Woodchopper

- Attach the resistance band to a stable anchor.
- Hold the handles with both hands and perform a diagonal chopping motion.

Benefit:

Engages the core, shoulders, and obliques.

Enhances functional movement patterns.

9. Tennis Ball

Exercise: Hand Squeezes

- Hold a tennis ball in your hand.
- Squeeze the ball and release, repeating the motion.

Benefit:

Strengthens hand and forearm muscles. Improves grip strength.

10. Balance Ball

Exercise: Wall Squats with Ball

- Place a stability ball between your back and a wall.
- Lower into a squat position while keeping the ball against the wall.

Benefit:

Strengthens the quadriceps, glutes, and improves posture.

When using small props, start with low resistance or intensity, and gradually progress. Ensure proper form and technique to prevent injury. Listen to your body and choose props that suit your fitness level and goals. Small props can add a dynamic element to your workouts while providing an enjoyable challenge.

Tips for a Safe and Effective Workout

Staying active is crucial for overall health and well-being, but it's important to approach exercise with safety in mind, especially for seniors. Here are some tips to ensure a safe and effective workout:

1. Consult with a Healthcare Professional:
Before starting any new exercise routine, consult with your healthcare professional, especially if you have pre-existing health conditions or concerns.

2. Start Slow and Gradual:
Begin with low-intensity exercises and gradually increase the intensity as your strength and endurance improve.

3. Warm-Up Properly:

Spend at least 5-10 minutes warming up with light cardiovascular activities like walking or marching in place to increase blood flow to your muscles.

4. Stay Hydrated:

Drink water before, during, and after your workout to prevent dehydration, which is essential for overall health.

5. Use Proper Equipment:

Wear comfortable and supportive footwear, and if using props or equipment, ensure they are in good condition and suitable for your fitness level.

6. Focus on Balance and Stability:
Incorporate exercises that improve balance and stability to reduce the risk of falls. Consider using a stable surface or chair for support if needed.

7. Listen to Your Body:
Pay attention to how your body feels during and after exercise. If you experience pain or discomfort, modify or stop the activity and consult with your healthcare professional.

8. Include Strength Training:
Incorporate strength training exercises to maintain muscle mass and support joint health. Start with light resistance and gradually increase as you become more comfortable.

9. Include Flexibility Exercises:

Stretching is crucial for maintaining flexibility. Include gentle stretching exercises to improve range of motion and prevent stiffness.

10. Practice Proper Breathing:

Focus on deep and controlled breathing during exercises. Proper breathing enhances oxygen intake and helps prevent dizziness.

11. Modify Exercises as Needed:

Tailor exercises to your individual needs. Use props or modify movements to accommodate any limitations or health concerns.

12. Cool Down:

Allow time for a proper cool-down after your workout to gradually lower your heart rate. Include gentle stretching to aid in muscle recovery.

13. Consistency is Key:

Aim for regular, consistent exercise. This helps maintain and improve physical function over time.

14. Socialize and Have Fun:

Consider joining group classes or exercising with friends to make workouts more enjoyable and social.

15. Stay Informed:

Stay informed about proper techniques and any modifications needed for your specific health conditions.

16. Stay Mindful:

Be present and mindful during your workout. Pay attention to your form and how your body responds to each movement.

17. Get Plenty of Rest:

Allow your body to rest and recover between exercise sessions. Quality sleep is essential for overall health.

Remember, it's never too late to start exercising, and incorporating these tips into your routine can help you enjoy the many

benefits of staying active in a safe and
effective manner.

Listening to Your Body

As we engage in physical activity, our bodies communicate with us, providing valuable feedback on our well-being and capabilities. Listening to these signals is crucial for a safe and effective workout, especially for seniors. Here's why it matters and how to tune in:

1. Avoiding Injury:
Paying attention to sensations like pain, discomfort, or unusual fatigue helps you identify potential issues before they escalate into injuries.

2. Understanding Limits:
Recognizing your body's limits prevents overexertion and allows for gradual progression in your fitness journey.

3. Customizing Workouts:

Everyone's body is unique, and listening to yours enables you to tailor exercises to your specific needs, ensuring a more personalized and effective workout.

4. Adapting to Changes:

Our bodies change over time, and being attuned to these changes allows you to adapt your workout routine to accommodate new needs or challenges.

5. Managing Health Conditions:

For individuals with pre-existing health conditions, listening to your body helps you navigate exercises that support your health without exacerbating underlying issues.

6. Recognizing Fatigue:

Understanding the difference between regular muscle fatigue and excessive exhaustion helps prevent burnout and promotes long-term consistency.

7. Improving Form:

Listening to your body cues you into proper form during exercises, reducing the risk of injury and ensuring targeted muscle engagement.

8. Promoting Mental Well-Being:

Paying attention to how exercise makes you feel emotionally and mentally is equally important. If a certain type of activity brings joy or relaxation, it contributes positively to your overall well-being.

How to Listen to Your Body:

1. Be Mindful:

Practice mindfulness during your workouts. Focus on the sensations in your muscles, joints, and overall energy levels.

2. Observe Pain vs. Discomfort:

Learn to distinguish between normal discomfort associated with challenging your body and pain that may indicate an issue. Pain is a signal to stop and reassess.

3. Monitor Breathing:

Pay attention to your breathing patterns. If you're struggling to breathe or experiencing dizziness, it may be a sign to take a break.

4. Stay Hydrated:

Dehydration can affect your performance and how your body feels during exercise. Stay hydrated to maintain optimal function.

5. Take Breaks:

Don't hesitate to take breaks when needed. Your body will thank you, and it helps prevent overexertion.

6. Adapt and Modify:

Be open to adapting exercises or modifying movements to suit your body's current capabilities. There's no one-size-fits-all approach.

7. Prioritize Recovery:

Allow sufficient time for recovery between workouts. Recovery is essential for muscle repair and overall well-being.

8. Consult with Professionals:

If you're uncertain about certain sensations or changes in your body, consult with healthcare or fitness professionals for guidance.

Listening to your body is a skill that improves with practice. It's a powerful tool for creating a workout routine that not only aligns with your fitness goals but also promotes overall health and longevity.

Consulting with a Healthcare Professional

Embarking on a new exercise journey is exciting, but it's essential to prioritize your health and safety. Consulting with a healthcare professional before starting any exercise program, especially as a senior, offers numerous benefits:

1. Personalized Assessment:

A healthcare professional can conduct a personalized assessment of your health status, taking into account any pre-existing medical conditions, medications, or potential risk factors.

2. Individualized Recommendations:
Based on your unique health profile, they can provide tailored recommendations for the type, intensity, and duration of exercise that best suits your needs and goals.

3. Identification of Risks:
Healthcare professionals can identify any potential health risks or contraindications that might impact your ability to engage in certain types of exercises.

4. Management of Chronic Conditions:
If you have chronic health conditions such as heart disease, diabetes, or arthritis, a healthcare professional can guide you on how to manage these conditions through appropriate exercise.

5. Safety Measures:

They can advise on safety measures, including any precautions you should take during exercise to minimize the risk of injury.

6. Medication Considerations:

Some medications may have side effects or interactions that can be influenced by exercise. Healthcare professionals can provide insights into how your medications might be affected.

7. Gradual Progression:

With their guidance, you can establish a plan for gradual progression, ensuring that you start at an appropriate level and progressively increase the intensity as your fitness improves.

8. Monitoring Vital Signs:

Regular monitoring of vital signs, such as blood pressure and heart rate, during exercise may be necessary. Healthcare professionals can guide you on what levels are safe for you.

What to Consider During Consultation:

1. Medical History:

Provide a comprehensive medical history, including any previous injuries, surgeries, or ongoing medical treatments.

2. Current Medications:

Share details about any medications you are currently taking, including dosage and frequency.

3. Lifestyle Factors:

Discuss your daily lifestyle, including stress levels, sleep patterns, and dietary habits, as these can impact your overall well-being.

4. Exercise Preferences:

Share your preferences and any previous experiences with exercise. This helps in creating a plan that you are more likely to stick with.

5. Goals and Expectations:

Clearly communicate your fitness goals and expectations, whether they involve weight management, improving mobility, or enhancing overall well-being.

6. Follow-Up Visits:

Establish a plan for follow-up visits to monitor progress, reassess your health status, and make any necessary adjustments to your exercise routine.

7. Communication with Fitness Professionals:

If you plan to work with a fitness professional, ensure that there is open communication between your healthcare provider and the fitness expert to create a collaborative and informed approach.

Remember:

Your healthcare professional is a valuable resource in creating a safe and effective exercise plan. Regular communication and updates with them ensure that your exercise routine aligns with your health goals and any changes in your health status.

Sample Wall Pilates Routines

Routine 1: Gentle Wall Pilates Flow

Warm-Up:

Standing Cat-Cow Stretch:

- Stand with your back against the wall.
- Inhale, arching your back away from the wall.
- Exhale, rounding your back and bringing your shoulders towards the wall.

Neck Stretch:

- Gently tilt your head from side to side, ear to shoulder, maintaining contact with the wall.

Core Activation:

Wall Sit with Pelvic Tilt:

- Slide down the wall into a seated position.
- Engage your core and perform gentle pelvic tilts.

Pilates Wall Exercises:

Wall Squats:

- Stand with your feet hip-width apart, back against the wall.
- Lower into a squat position, keeping your back against the wall.

Leg Lifts:

- Lie on your back with hips close to the wall.
- Lift one leg towards the ceiling, keeping the other bent.

Arm Reaches:

- Sit or stand with arms extended against the wall.
- Perform controlled arm reaches, engaging your core.

Cool Down:

Seated Forward Fold:

- Sit with your legs extended and lean forward, reaching towards your toes.

Chest Opener:

- Stand with arms bent at 90 degrees against the wall, opening your chest.

Routine 2: Balance and Flexibility Focus

Warm-Up:

March in Place:

- Stand with your back against the wall and march in place, lifting your knees gently.

Ankle Circles:

- Lift one foot and make circles with your ankle in both directions.

Balance and Stability:

Single Leg Balance:

- Stand on one leg, using the wall for support if needed. Hold for 15-30 seconds, then switch.

Heel-to-Toe Walk:

- Walk along a straight line, placing the heel of one foot directly in front of the toes of the other.

Pilates Wall Exercises:
Wall Plank:

- Face the wall and place your hands on it, then step back into a plank position.

Knee Lifts:

- Stand with your side to the wall, placing your hand on it.
- Lift your knee towards your chest, engaging your core.

Flexibility and Stretching:

Quad Stretch:

- Stand with your back against the wall, bend one knee, and bring your foot towards your buttocks.

Calf Stretch:

- Step one foot back, keeping the heel on the ground, and lean into the wall for a calf stretch.

Relaxation:

Seated Wall Meditation:

- Sit comfortably against the wall, close your eyes, and focus on your breath for 5 minutes.

Feel free to adjust the repetitions and durations based on your comfort level. If you experience any pain or discomfort, stop the exercise and consult with your healthcare professional. Enjoy your Wall Pilates routine!

15-Minute Daily Routine

Warm-Up (2 minutes):

March in Place (1 minute):

- Stand tall and lift your knees gently, marching in place.
- Swing your arms naturally to warm up the upper body.

Neck and Shoulder Rolls (1 minute):

- Slowly roll your shoulders backward, then forward.
- Gently tilt your head from side to side for neck mobility.
- Strength and Balance (5 minutes):

Wall Sit (1 minute):

- Slide down the wall into a seated position.

- Hold for one minute, engaging your core and thighs.

Leg Lifts (1 minute each leg):

- Lie on your back with hips close to the wall.
- Lift one leg towards the ceiling, then switch.

Chair Dips (1 minute):

- Use a stable chair or countertop.
- Lower your body by bending your elbows and then straighten.

Single Leg Balance (1 minute each leg):

- Stand on one leg, using the wall for support if needed.
- Focus on balance and stability.

Flexibility and Stretching (5 minutes):

Forward Fold (1 minute):

- Stand with feet hip-width apart and fold forward, reaching towards your toes.

Chest Opener (1 minute):

- Stand with arms bent at 90 degrees against the wall, opening your chest.

Seated Hamstring Stretch (1 minute):

- Sit with legs extended, reach towards your toes, keeping your back straight.

Quad Stretch (1 minute each leg):

- Stand with your back against the wall, bend one knee, and bring your foot towards your buttocks.

Calf Stretch (1 minute each leg):

- Step one foot back, keeping the heel on the ground, and lean into the wall for a calf stretch.

Relaxation and Cool Down (3 minutes):

Deep Breathing (1 minute):

- Sit or stand comfortably, close your eyes, and take deep, slow breaths.

Shoulder and Neck Release (1 minute):

- Gently roll your shoulders and tilt your head to release tension.

Seated Wall Meditation (1 minute):

- Sit comfortably against the wall, close your eyes, and focus on your breath.

Closing Thoughts:

This routine is a starting point, and you can adjust the durations or exercises based on your preferences. The key is to stay consistent and gradually increase intensity as you feel more comfortable. Remember to consult with a healthcare professional before starting any new exercise routine.

Customizing Your Workout

Customizing your workout is key to making it enjoyable, effective, and tailored to your individual needs and goals. Here are some tips on how to personalize your exercise routine:

Tips for Customizing Your Workout

1. Assess Your Fitness Level:

Begin by understanding your current fitness level. Assess your strengths, weaknesses, and any specific areas you want to target.

2. Define Your Goals:

Clearly outline your fitness goals. Whether it's improving flexibility, building strength, or enhancing overall well-being, having specific objectives will guide your customization.

3. Consider Your Preferences:

Identify the types of exercises you enjoy. If you like dancing, incorporate dance workouts. Enjoy nature? Consider outdoor activities like walking or hiking.

4. Account for Time:

Be realistic about the time you can dedicate to exercise. Customizing your routine to fit your schedule increases the likelihood of consistency.

5. Include Variety:

Keep things interesting by incorporating a variety of exercises. This prevents boredom and targets different muscle groups.

6. Listen to Your Body:

Pay attention to how your body responds to different exercises. Modify or eliminate movements that cause discomfort, and choose activities that feel good.

7. Adapt Based on Your Day:

Customize your workout based on how you feel each day. If you're full of energy, consider a more intense session. On lower-energy days, opt for gentle exercises.

8. Choose the Right Environment:

Whether you prefer the gym, home, or outdoor settings, pick an environment that motivates you. Your workout space greatly influences your overall experience.

9. Modify Intensity:

Adjust the intensity of your workout based on your energy levels. Some days you may push harder, while on others, a gentler approach may be suitable.

10. Incorporate Strength and Cardio:

Achieve a well-rounded workout by including both strength training and cardiovascular exercises. This promotes overall fitness and health.

11. Involve Functional Movements:

Include exercises that mimic daily activities. This enhances functional fitness, making everyday tasks easier.

12. Consult with Professionals:

Seek guidance from fitness professionals or healthcare providers. They can provide personalized advice and help tailor your routine to match your specific needs.

13. Progress Gradually:

If you're new to exercise or returning after a break, progress gradually. Build a solid foundation before increasing intensity or complexity.

14. Include Recovery Days:

Integrate rest and recovery into your routine. This allows your body to repair and reduces the risk of burnout or overtraining.

15. Track Your Progress:

Keep a record of your workouts. Tracking progress helps you celebrate achievements and identify areas for improvement.

16. Stay Hydrated and Nourished:

Hydration and proper nutrition play a vital role in your fitness journey. Ensure you're fueling your body adequately.

Customizing your workout is about making it uniquely yours. Tailor it to align with your preferences, goals, and lifestyle for a more enjoyable and sustainable fitness experience.

FAQs About Wall Pilates for Seniors

1. What is Wall Pilates?

Answer: Wall Pilates is a modified form of Pilates exercises that incorporates the support and stability of a wall. It involves using the wall as a prop to enhance body awareness, stability, and form during exercises.

2. Is Wall Pilates Suitable for Seniors?

Answer: Yes, Wall Pilates can be highly suitable for seniors. The support of the wall provides added stability, making it accessible for individuals with varying fitness levels. Always consult with a healthcare professional before starting a new exercise routine.

3. What Are the Benefits of Wall Pilates for Seniors?

Answer: Wall Pilates offers benefits such as improved posture, increased core strength, enhanced balance and stability, flexibility, and a gentle approach to overall fitness. It can be particularly beneficial for seniors looking for low-impact exercises.

4. Do I Need Special Equipment for Wall Pilates?

Answer: While some Wall Pilates exercises may use props like resistance bands or small balls, the primary equipment is a stable wall. No special or expensive equipment is necessary.

5. Can I Do Wall Pilates at Home?

Answer: Absolutely! Wall Pilates is adaptable to various settings, including home. All you need is a clear wall space. Ensure that the area is safe and free from obstacles.

6. How Long Should a Wall Pilates Session Last?

Answer: The duration of a Wall Pilates session can vary. For seniors, starting with shorter sessions, such as 15-30 minutes, and gradually increasing as comfort and fitness levels improve is a good approach.

7. Can Wall Pilates Help with Joint Pain?

Answer: Wall Pilates, with its emphasis on controlled movements and low-impact exercises, can be beneficial for individuals with joint pain. However, it's crucial to consult with a healthcare professional to ensure the exercises are suitable for your specific condition.

8. Is Wall Pilates Suitable for Beginners?
Answer: Yes, Wall Pilates can be suitable for beginners, including seniors who are new to exercise. Starting with basic movements and gradually progressing ensures a safe and effective introduction to Pilates.

9. Are There Any Safety Considerations for Wall Pilates?
Answer: Safety is paramount. Seniors should be cautious when getting up or down from the floor and ensure that the wall and surrounding area are free from hazards.

Consulting with a healthcare professional before starting is advisable.

10. Can Wall Pilates Help with Posture Improvement?

Answer: Yes, Wall Pilates emphasizes proper alignment and can contribute to improved posture. The exercises target core muscles, which play a crucial role in supporting good posture.

11. How Often Should I Do Wall Pilates?

Answer: The frequency can vary based on individual fitness levels and goals. Starting with 2-3 sessions per week and gradually increasing is a reasonable approach. Allow for rest days and listen to your body.

12. Can Wall Pilates Help with Balance and Fall Prevention?

Answer: Yes, Wall Pilates can be beneficial for improving balance and stability, contributing to fall prevention. However, individuals with specific balance concerns should consult with healthcare professionals for personalized advice.

Conclusion

In conclusion, Wall Pilates for seniors offers a gentle yet effective approach to improving overall fitness, balance, and flexibility. The support of the wall provides added stability, making it accessible for individuals of varying fitness levels. As with any exercise program, it's important to consult with a healthcare professional before starting to ensure that the routines are suitable for individual needs and health conditions.

The purpose of this guide is to empower seniors to embrace Wall Pilates as a part of their daily routine, emphasizing the numerous benefits it brings, including enhanced posture, increased core strength, and improved balance. By customizing workouts, incorporating a variety of exercises, and listening to the body, seniors can enjoy a safe and enjoyable fitness experience.

Remember, the journey to better health is a gradual process. Starting with shorter sessions and gradually increasing intensity, while being mindful of individual capabilities, ensures a sustainable and enjoyable fitness routine. Whether performed at home or in a fitness setting, Wall Pilates provides a versatile and adaptable approach to promoting overall well-being for seniors.

By incorporating the tips, exercises, and safety considerations outlined in this guide, seniors can embark on a fulfilling journey towards improved health, vitality, and a greater sense of well-being. Stay consistent, listen to your body, and enjoy the numerous benefits that Wall Pilates can bring to your daily life.

Here's to your health and happiness on this fitness journey!

Encouragement for Consistency

Congratulations on taking the first step towards a healthier and more vibrant you! Starting a fitness routine, like Wall Pilates, is a powerful decision, and I'm here to remind you that consistency is your superpower on this journey.

1. Embrace the Progress:
Every small step you take is progress. Whether it's holding a Wall Sit a bit longer or feeling a little more flexible, celebrate these victories. Progress may be gradual, but it's the consistency that makes it lasting.

2. Listen to Your Body:
Your body is unique, and it has its own language. Listen to it. If it says, "Let's push a

bit harder today," go for it. If it says, "I need a gentler approach," honor that too. It's a conversation, not a command.

3. Patience is Your Ally:
Rome wasn't built in a day, and neither is a stronger, healthier you. Patience is your ally. Trust the process, and remember that every consistent effort adds up over time.

4. Small Steps, Big Impact:
Consistency doesn't always mean big, drastic changes. It's the small, daily choices that create a ripple effect. A 15-minute Wall Pilates routine today can lead to a more energetic, resilient you in the future.

5. You're Worth It:

Taking time for yourself, investing in your well-being, and prioritizing your health are acts of self-love. You are worth every moment you dedicate to becoming the best version of yourself.

6. Celebrate the Journey:

The journey is just as important as the destination. Celebrate the joy in movement, the satisfaction of completing a session, and the newfound strength you discover within yourself.

7. Consistency Builds Habits:

Consistency isn't just about the exercises; it's about building healthy habits. As you make Wall Pilates a part of your routine, you're laying the foundation for a lifestyle that supports your well-being.

8. You've Got This:
On days when motivation wanes, remember why you started. You've got this, and the benefits awaiting you on the other side are worth the effort.

9. Reach Out for Support:
You're not alone on this journey. Reach out for support when needed. Share your successes, challenges, and experiences with others who are cheering you on.

10. Enjoy the Journey:
Most importantly, enjoy the journey. Wall Pilates isn't just about physical fitness; it's about the joy of movement, the discovery of

your body's capabilities, and the empowerment that comes with taking control of your health.

You're on a remarkable path, and your commitment to consistency is a testament to your resilience and determination. Keep going, keep growing, and remember that every step forward is a step towards a healthier, happier you.

With unwavering support,